MW01244612

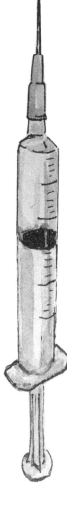

Welcome!

Article 7 of the International Covenant on Civil and Political Rights says, "...no one shall be subjected without his free consent to medical or scientific experimentation." True consent can not be given without informed consent.

In this era of misinformation and distrust, many people do not know where to start when learning about vaccines. Instead of giving answers, this book asks 50 questions for YOU to find the answers. Some answers are easy to find and others will take some digging. No source is off limits: ask doctors, nurses, medical researchers, the CDC website, studies published in the US National Library of Medicine, Children's Health Defense Science Library, online resources, and books. Research until you feel satisfied you have a deep understanding of the answer. Use the "notes" page to record any thoughts, quotes, statistics, or citations for your later reference.

We hope you enjoy this journey expanding your knowledge so you can make a truly informed decision for your family.

Yours,
Informed Consent Press

Notes:

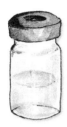

Question 1:

Name 7 Vaccine Ingredients:

1._____

2._____

3._____

4._____

5._____

6._____

7._____

Notes:

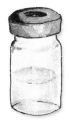

Question 2:

What is an adjuvant?

_____

_____

_____

_____

Notes:

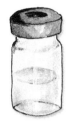

Question 3:

What is an antigen?

_____

_____

_____

_____

Notes:

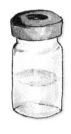

Question 4:

What is the National Childhood Vaccine Injury Act of 1986?

_____

_____

_____

_____

_____

_____

_____

_____

Notes:

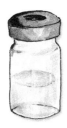 **Question 5:**

Can you sue the manufacturers of vaccines if your child is injured or dies?

☐ Yes

☐ No

Notes:

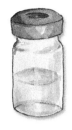

Question 6:

What is Vaccine Court?
How is Vaccine Court funded?

_____

_____

_____

_____

_____

_____

_____

_____

_____

Notes:

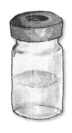

Question 7:

What is the National Vaccine Injury Compensation Program (VICP)?

_____

_____

_____

_____

_____

_____

_____

_____

_____

Notes:

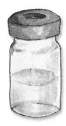

Question 8:

How much money has been paid out by VICP??

$ _____ , _____ , _____ , _____ .

Notes:

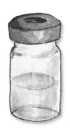 **Question 9:**

Who will take physical, emotional and financial responsibility for your child if they are injured?

_____

Notes:

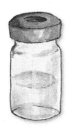

Question 10:

How many vaccine doses were in the CDC schedule between birth and age 18 when you were a kid?

_____

Notes:

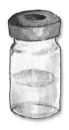

Question 11:

How many vaccine doses are in the CDC schedule between birth and age 18 now?

Notes:

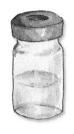

Question 12:

What is vaccine shedding?

_____

_____

_____

_____

_____

_____

_____

_____

Notes:

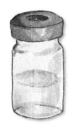

Question 13:

Can someone who was vaccinated for pertussis still spread pertussis, even if they show no symptoms?

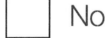 Yes

☐ No

Notes:

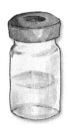

Question 14:

What was the death rate of people in the U.S. who likely contracted the measles BEFORE the vaccine was introduced in 1963?

☐ 0.01%

☐ 0.011%

☐ 0.012%

Notes:

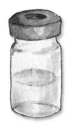

Question 15:

What does section 13.1 on the insert of every vaccine state?

_____

_____

_____

_____

_____

Notes:

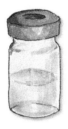

Question 16:

What is the rate of chronic
illness in children today?

Notes:

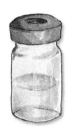

Question 17:

What is the current rate of autism?

1 in ___

What was it in 2000?

1 in ___

What was it in 1980?

1 in ___

Notes:

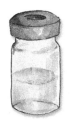

Question 18:

What happened when pediatric neurologist Andrew Zimmerman, the world-renowned pro-vaccine medical expert hired by the federal government to testify and win cases by debunking vaccine-autism claims in the secretive Vaccine Court, ended up coming to the conclusion that vaccines CAN cause autism in some children?

☐ *He was given a raise.*

☐ *He was sent on a press tour to raise awareness.*

☐ *He was immediately fired, his opinion was kept secret from other parents and the public, and the government misrepresented his opinion to continue to debunk vaccine-autism claims in Vaccine Court.*

Notes:

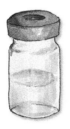

Question 19:

Who Said It?

"My name is _____ _____. I am a Senior Scientist with the Centers for Disease Control and Prevention, where I have worked since 1998. I regret that my coauthors and I omitted statistically significant information in our 2004 article published in the journal Pediatrics. The omitted data suggested that African American males who received the MMR vaccine before age 36 months were at increased risk for autism."

and

"I'm just looking at this and I'm like 'Oh my God....I cannot believe we did what we did...but we did [bury the data on these children]...It's all there...It's all there. I have handwritten notes.'"

Notes:

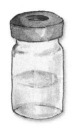

Question 20:

What is WI-38 and MRC-5?

Notes:

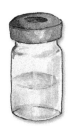

Question 21:

What is transverse myelitis?

_____

_____

_____

_____

_____

_____

_____

_____

Notes:

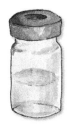

Question 22:

What is vaccine encephalopathy?
What are the symptoms?

_____

_____

_____

_____

_____

_____

_____

_____

_____

_____

Notes:

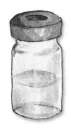

Question 23:

What is primary, secondary, and tertiary vaccine failure?

_____

_____

_____

_____

_____

_____

_____

_____

_____

_____

_____

_____

Notes:

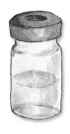

Question 24:

What is the difference between ingesting and injecting aluminum into your body?

Notes:

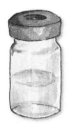

Question 25:

According to the FDA, what is an acceptable amount of aluminum to be injected into an infant?

_____

Notes:

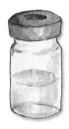

Question 26:

What is the aluminum content of the Hep B shot given at birth?

Notes:

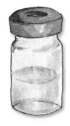

Question 27:

List the ways your baby can contract Hepatitis B:

_____

_____

_____

_____

Do you have Hepatitis B?

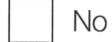 Yes

☐ No

Notes:

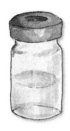

Question 28:

Define placebo:

_____

_____

_____

_____

_____

_____

_____

_____

Notes:

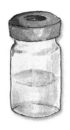

Question 29:

In the Gardasil (HPV) clinical trial, what ingredients were in the placebo control injection?

_____

_____

Bonus! What percentage of people receiving this "placebo" developed autoimmune issues?

☐ 2.1%

☐ 2.2%

☐ 2.3%

Notes:

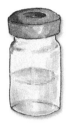

Question 30:

Name the vaccines that have been safety tested against an inert placebo control group:

_____

Notes:

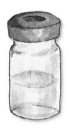 **Question 31:**

Do some vaccines contain dog,
monkey, pig, and human DNA?

☐ Yes

☐ No

Notes:

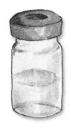

Question 32:

What is SV 40?

Notes:

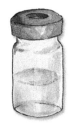

Question 33:

What is MTHFR and how is it affected by vaccines?

_____

_____

_____

_____

_____

_____

_____

_____

_____

_____

_____

_____

Notes:

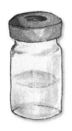

Question 34:

If your child has an adverse reaction to a vaccine, you should report it to VAERS. What does that acronym stand for?

_____ _____ _____

_____ _____

Notes:

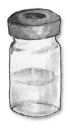

Question 35:

What is glyphosate?

_____

_____

_____

_____

_____

_____

Has it been found in vaccines?

☐ Yes

☐ No

Notes:

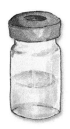

Question 36:

How many vaccine patents
does the CDC own?

Notes:

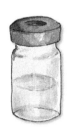

Question 37:

Who Was It?

After being the director of the CDC from 2002-2009, _____ _____ joined Merck to become their vaccine division president. In 2020, she sold $___ million worth of her stock in that company.

Notes:

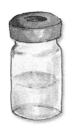

Question 38:

According to the 2010 U.S. Health and Human Services (HHS) pilot study by the Federal Agency for Health Care Research (AHCR), what ratio of vaccination resulted in reported injuries?

☐ 1 in 39

☐ 1 in 1,000

☐ 1 in 1,000,000

Notes:

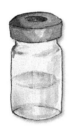

Question 39:

The CDC stopped responding to the researchers in the HHS pilot study when their data showed what percent of adverse vaccine reactions are currently being reported?

☐ 1%

☐ 30%

☐ 80%

Notes:

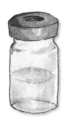

Question 40:

Who Said It?

"I think we cannot over-emphasize the fact that we really don't have very good safety monitoring systems... we're not able to give clear cut answers when people ask about the deaths that have occurred due to a particular vaccine."

- Dr. _____ _____, Chief Scientist at the World Health Organization, 2019

Notes:

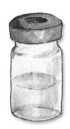

Question 41:

Treasure Hunt!

Find a study showing fully vaccinated vs fully unvaccinated health outcomes.

Notes:

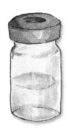

Question 42:

Treasure Hunt!

Find a safety study proving it is safe to inject multiple vaccines at once or a study proving the current schedule is safe.

Notes:

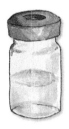

Question 43:

Treasure Hunt!

Find a study showing any vaccine has been tested on pregnant women and is safe for the unborn baby.

Notes:

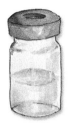

Question 44:

When Dr. _____ _____,
Vaccine Program Manager in
Nigeria, asked the World Health
Organization in December 2019,
"Has there ever been a study on
the possiblities of cross-reactions
of multiple antigens, adjuvants,
and preservatives from different
companies' vaccines given at the
same time?" the answer from the
WHO panel was:

☐ Yes

☐ No

Notes:

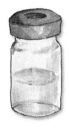

Question 45:

At your next doctor's appointment, ask your doctor the questions in this book. What did they score?

Are you satisfied with their knowledge?

☐ Yes

☐ No

Notes:

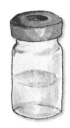

Question 46:

How much money does your doctor receive in bonuses from insurance companies and Medicaid for full compliance with the CDC vaccine schedule?

$ _____ , _____ .

Notes:

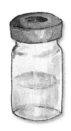

Question 47:

According to Prof. _____ _____, Ph.D., Professor of Anthropology and Director of the Vaccine Confidence Project, how much time is "a doctor lucky to receive in training on vaccines in medical school?"

☐ Half of a day

☐ 3/4 of a day

☐ One full day

Notes:

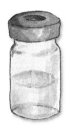

Question 48:

Homework Time!

Read Article 6 (Consent) in the UNESCO Universal Declaration on Bio-ethics and Human Rights. Then, fill in the blank:

The interests and welfare of the _____ should have priority over the sole interest of science or society.

Notes:

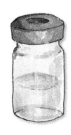

Question 49:

Name 10 ways to naturally boost your immune system.

1. _____
2. _____
3. _____
4. _____
5. _____
6. _____
7. _____
8. _____
9. _____
10. _____

Notes:

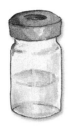

Question 50:

What are the three types of exemptions sometimes available for school children in the U.S.?

1. _____

2. _____

3. _____

Which exemptions are available in your state?

1. _____

2. _____

3. _____

Notes:

Extra Credit!

Who Said It?

"It is simply no longer possible to believe much of the clinical research that is published, or to rely on the judgment of trusted physicians or authoritative medical guidelines. I take no pleasure in this conclusion, which I reached slowly and reluctantly over my two decades as an editor of The New England Journal of Medicine."

– _____ _____, former editor-in-chief of the prestigious peer-reviewed medical journal, The New England Journal of Medicine

Notes:

Bonus Question!

What industry spends more than
TWICE as much as the oil and
gas industry in lobbying U.S.
elected officials?

_____

Notes:

Good job, Researcher!

Now that you have the answers to these questions, you are better informed to make your own choices about vaccinations. Whatever you decide, we wish you good health and a strong immune system!

ps: Don't let your research stop here! There are hundreds of other questions we could have included in this book.

Made in the USA
Middletown, DE
06 October 2022